To transplant patie[nts]
Remember, this j[ourney isn't all]
doom & gloom, there is hope for all
of us.
Stay healthy as you can.

Peace,
Jim
9/22/16

New Mountains to Climb

… a journey to lung transplant and beyond

Jim Carns

Single Lung Transplant

September 22, 2013

New Mountains to Climb

Foreword

Jim asked me to write this "foreword" a few months ago. I immediately agreed, then delayed doing so, fearing to mess up the task. Nudged by him, I'm trying again.

First of all, his is a story worth reading.

If you have been diagnosed with IPF, it will walk you through Jim's journey with this tough disease.

If your spouse, relative, or friend has IPF, you may be hungry to know what this diagnosis means for you, the caregiver. Front and center—your role is crucial.

I first heard a completely healthy Jim speak in public 15 years ago. He and Karen, leading a stewardship campaign, encouraged us all to reflect with gratitude on the gifts we had been given, and in turn how we could contribute to our community. When I next met Jim, he was in my office in the pulmonary clinic—I in the white coat and he completely pissed by the news that he needed to use oxygen. It was a major challenge to the "attitude of gratitude" he had worn so easily years earlier.

I now see Jim and Karen the last Monday of each month, from 5-7 pm, when Anne Dimmock convenes our local IPF support group in a conference room of the Penn State Hershey Fitness Center. We enter through a common area where lithe twenty something medical and nursing students pop in to buff their bodies, run their miles on the treadmills, and pump iron. Our group gathers for a different sort of work out. We push round tables together, greet familiar faces and catch up on the status of absent members.

Newcomers edge into the room, often shell-shocked by their diagnosis. Some bring oxygen tanks and a hacking cough. More than anything, they want to know what's ahead for them, or for their family member or friend. Our IPF support group walks with people through all the paths the IPF story brings—the periods of stability, the precipitous declines, the hospice, the successful transplant.

The central value of Jim's story is that it begins to answer the question "what is it like, really, to have IPF?" Sure, we all know that what happened to Jim might or might not happen to the next person with IPF. A minority of patients with IPF qualifies for, and has, a successful transplant. But Jim's story is a start to ending the utter isolation that often comes with an IPF diagnosis. More than anything I think Jim aims to end the isolation, and preserve community.

Last month, at support group, a newcomer proclaimed "I have IPF. It doesn't have me."

For Jim this is definitely true. I hear Jim's voice—his snarky humor, grim resolve, palpable relief, warm gratitude to Karen, and determination to give back, once again. He loves Karen, golf and Corvettes. Always has. Always will. So breathe. You are not alone. Despite this awful disease, Jim is still Jim. By extension, you will still be you. Phew.

As you may gather, Jim and his wife Karen have made an indelible impression on me. I commend his story to you.

- **Dr. Rebecca Bascom, MD**

About the Cover

As I was trying to pull this whole book together, I knew that I would need to have a cover that was eye catching and yet appealing to the reader. I looked at many dust covers on books, but nothing popped out at me. On December 25, 2015 I received that eye catching, yet appealing idea for my cover that I had been searching for.

As a Christmas present our granddaughter Alexis Iagnemma gave me the oil painting that you see depicted on the cover.

The painting means a lot to me, but the words on the bottom expresses much, not only to me, but I believe to many who will read this book.

Thanks Lex!

Love ya,

Peka

The Journey Begins

Imagine being told you have a disease you have never heard of, a disease with no known cause, for which there is no known effective medical treatment and no cure. Your future has been instantly shortened to three to five years. I want to share with you my journey with idiopathic pulmonary fibrosis (IPF).

Everyone's journey starts at birth; this is something I believe with all my heart. The beginning of my journey was not unlike millions of others. Born into a working class family, the youngest of three children, grew up in a small town, graduated from high school, got a job in the steel mill, got married, had three great kids, and got divorced.... Well, you get the idea.

In 1994 I remarried and have been extremely happy from that point on. Karen had not only become my wife, the love of my life and my best friend, but also in the past year or so my strongest supporter during my journey and, quite honestly, my caregiver. You see, in 2010 I was diagnosed with idiopathic pulmonary fibrosis.

In July of 2009 I became more aware of the fact I had a health problem. Karen and I were invited to go with friends to Colorado for a week of hiking and so-called relaxation. The first real indication I may have had a problem came when the doors of the airplane opened in Denver and I took my first deep breath of the "mile-high" air. When they say the air is thin, they aren't kidding!

I figured things had to get better when we arrived at our destination in Crested Butte. Boy was I wrong. It seemed like my breathing became more labored; maybe it was because we were at an elevation of almost 9,000 feet and sometimes higher. As long as I did not exert myself or hike the mountain trails, I was okay! Walking on level surfaces was not an issue, but not much hiking in Colorado is done on the level.

Hiking always found me bringing up the rear, and I don't mean I was hanging back to make certain no one got lost or injured on the way to the top of the mountain. To give you an example of how far back of the group I usually was, my friends passed me on their way back down the mountain as I was struggling to make it to the summit. This would not have been so bad if they had reached the top and turned around to come and see where I was, but they had the opportunity to have a snack and refresh themselves with an adult beverage or two. I will admit, once in a while they did check on me to make certain I was okay, but I told them I was fine and for them to be on their way. I think this was one of those ego things we hear so much about.

This trip to Colorado was the "slap upside my head" I needed to make me realize what I was experiencing was probably not normal. Up until this point in time, I had attributed what was happening to me to the fact I was 60 years old and probably not in the best shape of my life. I often joked with the people I was hiking with that they were trying to kill me, but looking back on this trip, I can probably say with all honesty they may have helped save my life.

Diagnosis

When we returned home, one of the first things I did was make an appointment with my primary care physician (PCP). After listening to my symptoms and giving me a complete physical, he determined I ought to see a cardiologist and have my heart checked. I had a battery of tests, X-rays, a heart catheterization, and it was determined my heart was strong and my heart was not the problem. I guess having the time to reflect on things, it may have been easier to correct a heart issue than to face what was to come. To this day, my heart is strong, and I have no known cardiac issues.

By mid-June 2010, a problem with my heart was ruled out, and despite what some people may think, they found I do have a heart, and it is quite healthy. My doctor strongly suggested I consider seeing a pulmonary specialist to check my lungs.

By the end of June, we, and by we I mean Karen and I, had my first of many visits to see a pulmonologist a Hershey Medical Center (HMC). There we saw Dr. Kevin Gleason. Karen has been by my side for this entire journey, to be honest I don't know how I would have made out if she had not been here to support me.

On June 25, 2010, I was diagnosed with interstitial lung disease, probably idiopathic pulmonary fibrosis.

What is idiopathic pulmonary fibrosis, you ask? As it was explained to us at this appointment, "IPF is an unpredictable, debilitating, and ultimately fatal disease, and there is no known cure. IPF has no known cause and affects about 70,000 people a year. This disease kills many patients within two to five years of diagnosis as progressive scarring of the lungs makes it impossible to breathe." Now, this appointment really put a damper on my entire day. How do I comprehend what I have isn't really going to go away and is probably going to kill me? There is no magic pill to take to cure this, and even a lung transplant is not a cure, nor is it a guarantee of survival.

What causes pulmonary fibrosis, might be the next question you ask? Well that is the million-dollar question. There is no known cause of this disease, at least nothing doctors or researchers can put their finger on at this time. In my case it could have been from smoking or maybe from working in the steel mill. Maybe it could be attributed to my yearlong vacation in Vietnam, but the VA doesn't agree with that possibility at the present time. Or how about the environment as a cause; we all know how dirty the air is. Maybe it could also be familial, and runs in my family, which means my kids, could possibly have the gene. The list goes on and on….

In my mind I needed more information about this disease; surely the doctors were wrong. Where else does one go to get good information? The Internet, of course! Boy, was that a mistake. One piece of advice I will share with you now is to stay off the Internet and leave the diagnosing, treatment, and answering of your questions to the medical staff that is treating you. I saw nothing on the Internet to make me feel good or lead me to believe I should even be alive at this point. Don't get me wrong, there are some good websites and some good information is available, but you must be very careful as to the information that is provided on the Internet. You are currently going to a doctor or soon will be seeking their advice. Stick with what they tell you and stay off the Internet.

For the next year we diligently went to scheduled appointments with various doctors and did pulmonary function tests (PFTs). What are pulmonary function tests, you ask? Well the short answer is they are noninvasive diagnostic tests that provide measurable feedback about the function of the lungs. By assessing lung volumes, capacities, rates of flow, and gas exchange, PFTs provide information, when evaluated by your doctor, can help diagnose certain lung disorders; i.e., pulmonary fibrosis. Our appointments were about every two to three months, and we were basically told the same thing: yes, you still have pulmonary fibrosis; no, there has still not been a breakthrough for a cure; and yes, your PFTs still show a slight deterioration, and let's try prednisone and see what happens. Well, nothing happened. I shouldn't say nothing happened; the prednisone did appear to help the nagging cough I had. The bottom line was I was stable, and my lung function was stable. When I started seeing the medical staff at the Hershey Medical Center, my lung capacity was 60%.

When the summer of 2011 arrived, we were still quite confused, and we were still searching for more information about pulmonary fibrosis. I was seriously considering going somewhere else for a second opinion.

My sister Ann became aware of an IPF conference that was going to be held in Harrisburg in September. This was the perfect opportunity for us not only to meet with others who were dealing with pulmonary fibrosis, but also hear what experts had to say about this disease. We registered, attended, and came away with a wealth of information and knowledge we did not have prior to this time. We met Dr. Paul Simonelli, another leading pulmonologist doing research on this disease as well as seeing patients who have been diagnosed with IPF. After talking with me, Dr. Simonelli agreed to see me and talk to us about pulmonary fibrosis.

I had no medical reason to disbelieve the original diagnosis. I just needed to be sure. In late October, I made an appointment at Geisinger Medical Center for this second opinion, where we met with Dr. Simonelli. My diagnosis was confirmed. I think I would recommend everyone get a second opinion, especially if there is doubt, other concerns, or you just want to reassure yourself you are doing everything possible.

Prior to my next appointment at Hershey, I received a call telling me my attending pulmonologist was no longer seeing patients. At this point in time I did have the option of being seen by Dr. Simonelli, who invited me to continue as one of his patients. I wasn't sure I wanted to travel an additional 50 plus miles to Geisinger, especially since HMC was only five miles from my home. This is just what we needed to add to our already high stress level. Should we go to Geisinger for treatment or remain at HMC?

We chose to stay at Hershey since my medical records are located there. After doing more research, I decided to get an appointment with Dr. Rebecca Bascom at HMC. Besides, it was closer to home, and as they say, the rest is history. Dr. Bascom has been on this journey with us since late in 2011.

In late October 2011 we met with Dr. Bascom, and had an extensive interview and exam. She concurred with the findings of my first and second opinion, and we agreed to start pulmonary rehab, consider supplemental oxygen usage, and prepare for the possibility of lung transplantation. I was also asked if I had an interest in participating in the pirfenidone drug study (more on this later), and of course it was suggested I return for a reassessment at regular intervals. At this point my lung capacity was down and probably would continue to drop even lower. The next six months or so were pretty uneventful. I had regular office visits with Dr. Bascom, PFTs, and of course, went back every three months for a follow-up visit.

One of my biggest annoyances or problems, and I probably shouldn't phrase it like that, throughout this whole ordeal has been going to an appointment and coming away feeling no better than I felt from the previous appointment, if that makes any sense. I guess I had expected or wanted to come away from each appointment or test with answers to this disease and with the hope I was getting better. I guess this is one of those "patience" things Karen thinks I need to continue to work on. It sounds like being back in the Army: hurry up and wait!

Up until this point things had been moving along at a slow but consistent pace, and unfortunately that slow pace continued downward. However, for the remainder of 2012 and for 2013 the pace of things picked up dramatically.

I started pulmonary rehab with PinnacleHealth in October 2012. I will admit I wasn't overly thrilled about going three times a week. It seemed to me I could probably get the same results at the gym and do it cheaper. One thing pulmonary rehab specialists did, I could not get done at the gym, was they put a monitor on me and kept tabs on my heart rate, oxygen level, EKG, and blood pressure. In this early leg of my journey, I was exposed to the fact I was going to need oxygen sooner rather than later.

They brought a long tube to me, and it was attached to the oxygen supply. This couldn't be happening to me, could it...? I don't need supplemental oxygen to live, do I? Do I need to use it all the time? What will the grandkids think? This development wasn't going over too well with me. I got home and told Karen what they did to me, and I literally broke down and cried. I didn't shed tears when I was diagnosed with IPF, but I sure did when they put me on supplemental oxygen at pulmonary rehab. After the initial shock wore off, I was able to accept the fact this bump in the road was necessary and helped me breathe easier.

When I had my next regular appointment with Dr. Bascom, we discussed my need or perceived need for oxygen. We all agreed I probably should use oxygen more, but Dr. Bascom reluctantly relented and told me if I could build up my strength and stamina, she would not insist I use supplemental oxygen 24/7 at this time. That was music to my ears. I agreed I would start doing more cardio activity on a regular basis to build up my lung strength and stamina. I think I would have made a deal with the devil to avoid using oxygen.

I became a mall walker and found I was not the only one using the mall for exercise. I came to find out I became member of a group that walks the mall for various health reasons. The deal I made with Dr. Bascom about doing more cardio exercise didn't last long. In late spring of 2013, it came to pass I would need to use oxygen on more or less a regular basis, especially with any type of physical exertion.

Along with Dr. Bascom, we talked at length, about the pirfenidone drug study I was asked to consider and possibly participate in. On November 12, 2012, I started participating in this study. My participation was supposed to last one year. It was a blind study, and to be honest, I had nothing to lose. Pirfenidone is an experimental drug that has not yet been approved for use in the states but has been approved in Europe, Japan, and Canada. Pirfenidone is supposed to reduce the rapid decline in lung function. I knew this drug would probably never benefit me, but maybe, just maybe, it could provide relief or help find a cure for somebody sometime in the future. I also figured this would be another level of care that would or could be available to me, and I would have a doctor keeping tabs on me between my regular appointments. In the blind study, I was not supposed to know if I was being given the real drug or a placebo. It only took until springtime 2013 for me and the doctors to figure out I was probably taking the real drug instead of a sugar pill. Some of the side effects, and thankfully they were minor, were sensitivity to the sun and an annoying rash on areas being exposed to the sun. I participated in this drug study until the time of my transplant.

Preparing for Transplant

I returned to HMC for scheduled PFTs and appointments. In late November 2012 the suggestion was strongly made that I ought to make certain I have my affairs in order, pick a transplant hospital to work with, and at least have the initial introduction made so we might begin the transplant evaluation process.

Another reason we thought it would be best to start the evaluation process now rather than later was the fact that we knew with IPF my health could remain steady for a long period of time, but we also knew with this disease my health could possibly take a significant nosedive in a short period of time, and then it is often too late to start the evaluation process.

WOW. This was a huge step for us, not totally unexpected, but still a huge step nonetheless. Fortunately for us, or I guess I should say me, I had started doing my research knowing this day would sometime present itself, and I wanted to be in the best hands available.

I was aware one of the leading transplant surgeons in the country was Dr. Yoshiya Toyoda, and he was leading the transplant team at the University of Pittsburgh Medical Center (UPMC), which also happens to be one of leading transplant facilities in the United States. So this, we thought, made my decision easy: We would be running the turnpike heading west to Pittsburgh. This is one decision we had out of the way.

After we thought my selection was solid and we were ready to move forward and make necessary appointments with the doctors and medical staff at UPMC, Karen and I found out Dr. Toyoda had left that facility and was now heading the lung transplant program at Temple University Hospital in Philadelphia. Okay, this was another small bump in the road. Instead of heading west to Pittsburgh on the Pennsylvania Turnpike, we will be changing course and heading east to Philadelphia. I still want the best surgeon and surgical team available to do my surgery if and when it is time.

Dr. Bascom made the initial appointment, and we met with Dr. Francis Cordova on December 20, 2012, at Temple University Hospital in

Philadelphia. Dr. Cordova would be my transplant physician during this part of my journey.

We first met with Transplant Coordinator, Debbie Doyle. Debbie explained to us the process that would be required to even be considered for transplant. She told us if Dr. Cordova agreed I should be considered for transplantation, I would be required to come to Temple for almost two weeks of testing. She related that when the testing was completed, I would know more about myself than I could ever imagine, and, boy, was she right. She gave us a large three-ring binder that had everything imaginable about the evaluation and the transplant process.

Dr. Cordova came in and did a cursory exam and looked at the x-rays and scans we had brought with us from previous testing and doctors' visits at HMC and Geisinger Medical Center. Dr. Cordova appeared to be less than convinced I should be there, and in his opinion I was too healthy to be considered for transplant. It almost seemed to us he was testing us to see if we really knew what we were talking about when it came to this disease and if we knew what we could or would be getting ourselves into.

I agreed with Dr. Cordova that I was probably healthier than a lot of other patients with IPF who were waiting for a transplant. We made our case that we were well aware that currently I was on a slow decline as far as my lungs and breathing were concerned. We discussed that with this disease my health could continue deteriorating slowly for quite some time, but I was also quite aware that drastic changes could occur at any time, and at that point it could possibly be too late to be considered for lung transplantation.

Like I said previously, I believe this meeting could have been a test, and it appeared we passed. Dr. Cordova agreed, maybe reluctantly, but he did agree I should proceed with the transplant evaluation process.

On January 27, 2013, the next leg of this journey was to begin. We wondered why it took over a month to start this evaluation process. It appears that sometimes things move slower than one anticipates... again; it was that patience thing Karen kept telling me I needed to work on. I understood they had to check my insurance to make certain they would be paid for all services and I would not be surprised by any unanticipated expense. It was also pointed out it takes time to schedule all of the necessary testing and doctor's visits that would be required.

A week or so prior to my first appointment at Temple, we had a call from the social worker at Temple, and she wanted to know if she could be of help getting us a place to stay while I was going through the evaluation process. To be honest, I don't think Karen or I even thought that far ahead. She suggested the Gift of Life Family House (GOLF House) and offered to make the introduction since we had to be referred to them by the hospital. I will tell you more about this facility later.

We received a detailed schedule from the Temple Lung Center telling me where I was supposed to be, when I was supposed to be there, and what they were going to do to me. Starting on January 28 at 7:00 a.m., I was supposed to be there for registration, and not only did I get registered, but the lab people also drew 22 vials of blood from me for different types of screening and testing.

Between January 28 and February 27, we had meetings with doctors, nurses, surgeons, psychologists, nutritionists, cardiologists, speech pathologists, and social workers. Also during this period I was poked, prodded, and jabbed in various ways and places. I had tests coming out the old wazoo! I had CAT scans, chest X-rays, EKGs, echocardiograms, a tine test to make certain I didn't have TB, pulmonary function tests, six-minute walk, a muga scan, a maximum exercise test, psychological testing, lung scan, DEXA scan, Dopler study, heart catherization, barium swallow, and probably a few other tests I can't recall or probably don't want to recall.

All of the tests were performed on various days at Temple. Some of the days I had several tests and meetings with doctors, and then on other days it was just one test or appointment. None of the tests I completed would deter me from the decision to move forward with a possible transplant. I will admit the time I spent at the hospital did tire me out, and each night I was anxious to get back to the GOLF House to eat and go to bed. It definitely made for long days for me, but I really believe the days must have seemed much longer for Karen, who waited patiently in the waiting room while I was having tests.

Out of all of these tests I endured, the only deficiency they found with me besides my lungs was that I supposedly had an abscess in one of my rear molars. I had always thought if you had an abscess in one of your teeth, it would hurt like h***. When I got home, it was off to my dentist, and after more X-rays I was told what they were seeing was a shadow from a root canal I had done 30+ years ago. Temple was satisfied with that explanation, and the case was closed.

As I mentioned earlier, Temple did arrange for us to stay at the GOLF House while we were in Philadelphia during this time. The GOLF House is similar to the Ronald McDonald House in Hershey, only this house is used for patients and families who are in town for doctors' appointments at one of the six area transplant hospitals in Philadelphia. The GOLF House became a home away from home for us after long days of testing at Temple. We were able to go back to the GOLF House and relax, get a hot meal, and talk to others who were experiencing the same issues as we were. It gave us someone to talk to and gain more information pertaining to this journey we were on. Some of the people were there because they were going through the same evaluations I was. Some people had had transplants and were in town for follow-up appointments. Some were families who were there because they had someone in the hospital who had received a transplant, and there were people at the GOLF House who were there waiting for an organ to become available so they could receive a transplant and a second chance at life.

Early in March 2013, we received a letter from the transplant team letting us know if I would or should be listed for transplant at this time. They had determined at the present time I was not sick enough to be put on the transplant list. On one hand, this decision was a disappointment to us, but on the other hand, this decision probably was the correct one to be made at that particular time, and it really was not unexpected. The main thing we wanted to accomplish was to get this evaluation process out of the way or at least started in case my condition deteriorated more rapidly than anticipated. We were aware some of these tests may need to be repeated at some point in time, but the majority of the tests would be out of the way. They wanted me to return in May for a follow-up appointment.

My appointment on May 16 came and I did my PFTs and six-minute walk before seeing Dr. Cordova. During this meeting Dr. Cordova told us it was probably time to get me listed. We assume my PFTs and six-minute walk numbers were not very good and he would recommend to the transplant team I be put on the list.

On May 28 the transplant team met, and on June 10, I received a letter from Temple stating that because of my diagnosis of "end stage pulmonary fibrosis" I was being put on the active list for lung transplantation. I would need to be seen by Dr. Cordova every four to six weeks so my condition could be monitored more closely. I said previously that when I was diagnosed with IPF it put a damper on my day, but when I got the letter stating "end stage pulmonary fibrosis," that really hit me hard. The words "end stage" to me meant that whatever was going to happen would be sooner rather than later. At this point of my journey, I was in the hands of God and the medical staff at Temple University Hospital.

We were told my Lung Allocation Score (LAS) was a relatively low score and not to expect anything to happen for quite some time, probably at least six months or more. The LAS is a numerical value used by the United Network for Organ Sharing (UNOS) to assign relative priority for distributing donated lungs for transplantation within the United States. The LAS score takes into account various measures of a patient's health, the reason for all the transplant evaluation testing I did earlier, in order to direct donated organs toward the patients who would best benefit from a lung transplant.

My next appointment was on August 15, and everything was status quo and nothing new had developed with my lungs since I was listed in June; at least things were not rapidly deteriorating. As we were wrapping up my appointment and small talk was being made, Karen and I told Dr. Cordova we wanted to go on a trip to Alaska in the summer of 2014, and I jokingly suggested maybe they could get off their a$$'s and move this process along.

I had an appointment with Dr. Arnold Meshkov, who is now my cardiologist, on September 12 and was not to return to see Dr. Cordova until October 3.

Little did I know what was going to happen in the upcoming weeks!

It was difficult for us to make plans to do anything. Since I had been listed for transplant, we had been limited in our travels; we had to pretty much stay in a three-hour radius of Temple. Anytime we went anywhere, we had to be prepared in case we got the call. Karen had her "transplant" bag packed at all times, just in case. I, on the other hand, well, I really wasn't going to need much, at least initially. What I needed was going to be provided to me - that sexy little hospital gown! Of course, I did make certain I had a couple of pairs of shorts, t-shirts, and slippers. I can't say the same for Karen. I must admit she was well prepared for when the call came. She had a list of things she needed to gather from each room in the house to take with her for her part of this journey. On the other hand, everything I needed would fit neatly into a brown paper bag.

Since my last appointment, everything was moving as it had been. I was still walking as much as I could and was still on two-three liters of oxygen and still getting tired very quickly. Carrying the oxygen bottle around when I was walking became a pain in the rear. A friend suggested I go to Wal-Mart or some place and get a hydration type backpack to carry the bottle around. It was more comfortable and much easier to carry around, and the small oxygen bottles fit in it quite nicely.

Since we really couldn't go anywhere, we decided now would be the time for us to have hardwood floors installed in the house. We had the flooring delivered on September 20, and they were to begin the installation on Monday, September 23. As they say, good idea... but the timing was not so good!

The Call

Temple University Hospital – 9/22/2013 – 09/30/2013

On the morning of September 22, we were getting ready for church; in fact, we were just about ready to walk out the door to go pick up our granddaughter, as we do on most Sundays. About 7:15 a.m., my cell phone rang, and Karen answered it. The voice on the other end was Debbie Doyle from the Temple Lung Center, who told Karen, "This is the call you are waiting for." They had a lung, and the procurement team was on its way to check it out, and if the lung was healthy and viable, they wanted me at the hospital as soon as we could safely get to Philadelphia.

Karen told me of the call, and all different emotions hit me at once. There was excitement, knowing what we have been waiting for could be close at hand; apprehension, knowing for what I was about to go through there were no guarantees whatsoever the transplant was going to be successful; even a twinge of sadness and guilt knowing while we were pretty excited, we also knew another family was grieving at this very same time.

Karen and I had our moment together in the kitchen; we held each other, tried to reassure each other everything was going to be alright, shed a tear or two, and I am sure we each said a prayer.

My sister Ann was the next call to be made. Ann was going to be Karen's support person during this part of my journey. Knowing Ann is not a morning person, I thought it was only fair I give her a little extra time to pack and get herself ready. I told her we would pick her up in 20 minutes. When we got there she was standing in the driveway, ready to go; this was probably the quickest she was ever ready to go anywhere.

Karen was packed and ready to go for the most part, and it didn't take me long to put my few things in that brown paper bag I had talked about earlier. Karen had packed her travel bag the night before because we were planning to go on a car cruise with our Corvette friends later on Sunday. After a last look around the house, by 7:35 a.m. we were on our way to pick up Ann.

One thing Karen was quite good at, and we thought very important, was to be prepared and ready to go when that call came, no matter what time of day or night it was. That bag was always packed and at the ready. When the call comes, that is not the time to be trying to decide what needs to be packed.

I knew I had to call our kids and tell them what was happening, and even if this turned out to be a dry run, they needed to know. These calls were difficult for me to make. I know I added additional worry for them, but I also had to do it for my own peace of mind. You never know....

An observation I have made since my transplant and I certainly believe this, prayer does work. Before we even got to the hospital and definitely prior to my being wheeled into the operating room, our granddaughter and Ann's husband Jim, had told the ministers at our Church that we got "the call" and were on our way to Philadelphia. Our ministers asked the congregation to keep us in their thoughts and prayers. Not only were we on the prayer list at our home church, but because of the extensive telephone and email list Karen had put together, we were on the prayer lists of several churches in the Harrisburg area and in the thoughts and prayers of many of our friends. Prayer does work, and God does listen.

Our drive to the hospital was uneventful. In fact, Ann remarked that she could not believe how at ease and peaceful Karen and I appeared to be. I think the reason was we knew what we were going to do when the call came. There was no second guessing this decision; our decision was made, and we were comfortable with it. We were quite aware what the risks were and we were looking forward to all of the positive benefits we believed were going to follow the successful transplant procedure. Don't get us wrong, deep down, and especially in me, we were plenty scared.

The Transplant

We were at Temple by 10:00 a.m. As we were told by Debbie, when we got the call, they would be expecting me at the Admissions Office. When we arrived, the nurse greeted me by saying, "You must be our Mr. Carns." After signing papers, we were off to the third floor to be prepped for surgery. We got to the surgical floor, and they had me put on one of those sexy hospital gowns I had been talking about, gave a urine sample, gave some more blood, and of course signed a few more papers. Karen and I had a few minutes to ourselves before they had me get on a gurney and rolled me down the hallway to the operating room. I know I said previously making those calls to the kids was difficult, but the most difficult time I had this day was watching Karen as they took me away and rolled me toward the operating room. We knew there were risks, and we knew in the back of our minds something could go wrong. Thankfully that was something neither of us had to worry about.

I was in the operating room by 11:00 a.m., and the nurses and doctors were talking to me about the operation. As soon as they were confident the donor lung was in good condition and was suitable for me, special IV lines were attached, and I was put to sleep by the anesthesia team. The last I remember looking at the clock on the wall it said 11:05 a.m., and that is the last thing I remember until I woke up in the intensive care unit.

Dr. Akira Shiose was the magician and surgeon who performed my single lung transplant.

I was told this is how the events for the remainder of the day unfolded: Once my donor lung had arrived at Temple and the transplant team deemed it suitable, the chest was opened and preparations were made to remove the old lung. The left lung was removed, and the new lung was stitched in place. This was done by sewing together the ends of the airway and main blood vessels leading in and out of the lung. After ensuring the new lung was working well, my chest was closed, leaving chest tubes to drain any blood or fluid that might otherwise accumulate around the new lung. Sounds like a piece of cake!

From what I understand, my surgery lasted approximately five or six hours. When the surgery was completed and all the doctors and nurses were done admiring their handiwork and patting each other on the back, I was taken to the intensive care unit. I think they just wanted a chance to admire a job well done.

I remember waking up in the ICU; I believe it was sometime on Monday. Karen tells me it was in the morning and my arms were strapped so I couldn't move, I assume so I could or would not do any harm to myself or rip any of the various tubes out of my body. The nurse said if I could behave and not pull my tubes or IVs out, they would release my arms. I quickly agreed to her requests. I tried talking to the nurse, but it was difficult because I had a breathing tube down my throat; fortunately we were able to communicate.

It wasn't long before they removed the breathing tube and I was breathing with my new lung. What an odd feeling, I would say it was almost surreal. I was a little apprehensive when they removed the breathing tube; in fact, you could say I was scared. I actually was breathing without the help of supplemental oxygen and I was not gasping for air. What a great feeling! I was actually breathing with a healthy lung, and now it was going to be up to me to take care of it.

I remember Karen being with me in the ICU, and I told her how pretty the walls were and I bet it took them a long time to paint because of all the paisley and psychedelic designs. They sure were pretty walls! I came to find out the walls were hospital white, and they were not painted. I was seeing these designs because of the drugs, and I probably was hallucinating. This was not the only time I saw pretty colors and designs on the walls at the hospital: when they moved me upstairs to my room, those walls were sometimes painted with those same pretty colors and designs. I really don't remember much of what happened this day, but I do remember the conversation about the walls with Karen. I've come to learn the drugs transplant patients are given affect each of us differently until the medical staff gets them adjusted properly. Hallucinations are not uncommon; some are good, like the ones I was having, but others were more nightmarish and hard to control.

I was told I was going to be moved to the sixth floor of the main part of the hospital as soon as a room became available; there I would be surrounded by other transplant patients and a specialized medical staff. I am not sure what time of the day they told me this, but I wasn't moved until late Monday evening or very early Tuesday morning.

My Post-Operative Experiences

I think I was just getting settled in the room, enjoying the paint on the walls, when it was time to get up for the day. Days start early at Temple, 6:00 a.m. to be exact. They come in and want to know how you feel or if you need help bathing. I wonder what they really expected me to say other than, "I feel like crap and I just came from the ICU and I really would appreciate some help getting cleaned up. After all, you have me hooked up to so many wires and tubes it is difficult for me to even move, let alone do anything for myself."

Each morning for the next week started off pretty much the same way. After the initial chorus of, "Time to get up," they come in and take your blood pressure, temperature, draw blood, do an EKG, I can't forget the X-rays and change the linens on the bed. Today, since I had come to the floor in the middle of the night, there was no breakfast for me. It seemed like an eternity until somebody decided I might be hungry and should have something to eat. Keep in mind the last time I ate was probably Saturday evening, and it was now Tuesday morning, and a lot had happened since then.

The nurses had to get a doctor to authorize a meal for me so I could eat. In the meantime the nurses and physical therapist thought it was time I got up and went for a walk. With their help I was able to walk to the nurse's station across the hall right outside my door, probably no more than 30 feet. Success, but I couldn't have done it without their help, and it really played me out!

Now my 40-day odyssey with food started.... I understand they wanted to make certain whatever I swallowed went into my stomach and not into my lungs.

It is my understanding Dr. Cordova authorized me to be on a regular diet and ordered a plate of the finest hospital fare to be delivered to my bedside. Now we are getting somewhere, I thought. By mid-morning I had some food, not sure what it was, but when you are hungry you will eat just about anything. I was enjoying the meal as much as I could, until Lauren Ciniglia, the Speech Therapist, came bouncing in and wanted to know what I was doing and who authorized this food. In my mind it should have been pretty obvious to her what I was doing, but not wanting to pi$$ anybody off my first day on the floor, I answered her questions. Obviously my answers were not the correct ones because she told me Dr. Cordova shouldn't have ordered this meal for me, so she picked up my tray and took it away and said she would get me something else to eat.

She brought me another tray and the food was pureed! Now, I don't know if you ever were on a pureed diet, but I can assure you there is nothing more disgusting looking or unappetizing than seeing a scoop of various colors on your plate and not knowing what it is or was and then having someone expect you to eat it. Add to this pureed diet the fact any liquid I wanted must have "thicken" in it, thickened to the consistency of honey. The speech therapist informed me I would be on this diet until I had a barium swallow test done and they were satisfied I had no issues with swallowing. I understood the speech therapist was only doing her job trying to make sure all food and liquids go into my stomach and do not end up in my new lung.

What is a barium swallow test? It is a radiologic examination of the swallowing function that uses a special movie-type X-ray called fluoroscopy. The patient is observed swallowing various types of substances that can be seen by fluoroscopy (usually liquid barium and/or foods coated with barium) in order to evaluate his or her ability to swallow safely and effectively. Patients are often observed swallowing various consistencies and textures, ranging from thin barium to barium-coated cookies. This exam is often performed with a speech-language pathologist present and until I passed this test, I can't have solid food. It was not until right before Thanksgiving I was able to pass this test and taken off this restrictive diet.

This was all done prior to the doctors being in to see me when doing their rounds. I figured the way my day had been going so far, the doctors would not have much good news to tell me.

The surgeon, Dr. Shiose, was in and was quite pleased with my recovery so far. He suggested to me they would try and have me out of the hospital within two weeks. That sounded pretty good to me because we were expecting a hospital stay of three to five weeks total. Dr. Shiose also said they would be taking out one of the drainage tubes that afternoon. After that tube was removed, I still had one more drainage tube and the catheter to get rid of. I will admit, after the surgeon left the room, my day did brighten somewhat, but I was still hungry!

19

Karen and Ann were with me the rest of the day. I don't think I ever realized how nice it was to have familiar faces around you when you are in strange surroundings, especially if you are not certain what is going to be happening. Like I said, it is good to see some familiar faces, but also you don't really like to have people see you at your worst, and I believe this was pretty much the worst for me.

Wednesday started just like the day before did. I have to make another admission here: I can say I never felt as helpless in my life as I was after the surgery. I literally could not do the things I normally did prior to my surgery, like bathe myself and go to the bathroom. I think it was a combination of feeling helpless and embarrassed. Enough said about this subject.

The doctors were in; again, they were pleased with my progress so far. They said they were going to remove the catheter today, and they alluded to the fact I could be discharged after only 10 or 11 days in the hospital. That sounded pretty good to me, but I certainly didn't want them to rush things just to free up a bed.

The physical therapist came in, and he had me out of bed and walking the halls. It seemed strange that something I would have done a few days before now turned into a real chore. When Karen came for the day, we walked the halls some more. I was happy I could do one lap, but that lap quickly tired me out. The doctors did tell me this was normal and I would feel the effects of this surgery for months to come.

Before the doctors moved on to the next patient, they told me a barium swallow had been ordered for today, but it had to be cancelled because I had been given morphine the prior evening and the doctor said I could not have any drug of this type in my system prior to this test. Surely you would have thought someone would have read my chart and this would have been noted.

Once again Karen and Ann were with me throughout the day. I feel certain that being in the hospital room with me made for an extremely long day for them. For me, though, since I wasn't going anywhere quite yet, I surely enjoyed having them around. I tried to make certain they got back to the GOLF House before dark so they could get some rest and a good meal

Thursday started just like the other days; up at 6:00 a.m.; the nurse came in to see if I needed help with anything, got me out of bed so they could change the linens, and wanted to know if I wanted to take a bath and get cleaned up. The answer was yes, but this time I didn't want help; I wanted to do it myself. Believe it or not, this was difficult, but to be quite honest I didn't want anybody else doing what I could be doing for myself.

Breakfast came, but there was something different this time; I had the usual oatmeal, applesauce, and pudding, but there was something else on my tray. My meds were there in "pill" form. They wanted to stop giving me my meds intravenously. The only problem with this was I needed to take the pills one at a time, and I needed to mix them with pudding or applesauce so they were easier for me to swallow. If I only had one pill to take it probably wouldn't have been so bad, but taking what seemed to be a whole handful was a different story altogether. I certainly am glad this wasn't a contest. It appeared to me it probably would have been easier to give a pet a pill than to get a patient weaned from taking drugs intravenously to taking drugs in pill form. Oh well, it helped me pass the time.

They did have me scheduled for the barium swallow on this day. Soon after breakfast they came and wheeled me down to the basement for this test. The fluoroscope must have been out of whack because they told me I was still having difficulty swallowing and they wouldn't approve me for a regular diet. I had to disagree with them, but they didn't want to listen to me. I would need to remain on this pureed diet until I had another test.

The nurses did allow me to have four pieces of chipped ice at a time, as long as I had a responsible adult with me while I sucked on these ice chips. I wanted to know when this barium swallow test would be scheduled again. As you might imagine, I was quite anxious to pass this test and get this barium swallow behind me. The doctors said it would be sometime the following week because the hospital could only do it twice in the same week because of my insurance coverage. I figured this would probably work out since I anticipated I would still be a guest here at Temple, and it would give me something to look forward to and break up the monotony.

I was back in my room before the doctors made their rounds, or maybe they had already been by and they were making a return trip. Although I was sort

21

of down in the dumps because of the swallow test, the doctors did give me some good news: they were going to remove the final drainage tube on this day. This means I was almost tube free. The only tube I had left was the port in my arm they have been giving me my drugs through. They really haven't been using it much since I started taking my meds orally. Once again taking drugs orally sounds easy and something else we normally would take for granted.

Our daughter Jenny came to visit today to make certain what she had been hearing about my recovery was factual. I suppose I also would have some doubts about an operation as major as the one I just went through. We had a good visit and I was able to convince her that I was going to be ok. Seeing faces of family is good medicine. Jen's visit also served a dual purpose. When she left, she took my sister back to Harrisburg so that they both can resume some sort of normal life.

Karen and I walked the halls quite a bit this afternoon. I found myself getting stronger with each passing day, and I was determined I was going to do everything I could to make this operation a success. The gift I received was too valuable not to take care of.

Friday arrived just like any other day. It started with the charge nurse coming in at 6:00 a.m. to see what kind of help I might need. The doctors came around, and again they were quite pleased with how my recovery was progressing. They checked the wounds, and they were healing nicely; the lung was strong and the X-rays had shown no sign of rejection up to this point, and everything still appeared to be attached just like they were on Sunday. In fact, the doctors hinted they might release me on Monday.

Wow, that sure was great news; in fact, I thought they may have been talking about one of the other patients. Nope, they said it was me, and as long as no complications occurred and the physical therapist thought I could reasonably take care of myself at home, understood my restrictions, and had my drug regimen down pat, they thought I could be released as long as I had a responsible adult to help me. I vouched for Karen, and they approved.

I was so excited; I could hardly wait for Karen to get there so I could share the good news with her. This day she was late getting to the hospital.

Although she had some needed "me" time, she was waiting for our daughter to get there. Linda was coming to spend a couple of days with her mom and visit with me.

Another highlight of my stay at "Hotel Temple" was when I told Karen and Linda I couldn't wait to get out so I could wash my greasy, dirty hair. Karen and Linda said they would do it for me, but now the question became: how? The nurses said they use a dry shampoo cap that has little or no water involved. It was heated in a microwave, the cap was put on my head, massaged into my scalp, and then I had to sit there with this stupid hat on. This was one of those Kodak moments they took advantage of. Thank goodness those pictures did not show up on Facebook. We all had a good laugh over this.

Also, that evening Linda helped to get us online, and we Skyped with the grandkids in Wisconsin and the next day we were going to Skype with the Virginia kids. This was good for all of us, and I think the kids were a little more relieved to see I was making such good progress with my recovery.

Saturday and Sunday came in just like the other days, up at 6:00 a.m., vitals checked, bathed, linens changed, and I was plopped into my chair to await breakfast and the doctors to make their rounds. It appears the hospital goes into slow motion when the weekend rolls around. I in no way mean to say I wasn't cared for, but it just seemed so much more relaxed. The doctors I had seen all week were nowhere to be found; instead they had fellows, interns, and residents doing the rounds. I feel certain their work and findings were being closely monitored by the doctors. When they came in and checked me, they kept saying how impressed they were with my recovery. To be honest, they were the same doctors or soon-to-be doctors who had been shadowing my pulmonary doctors and surgeon all week. They confirmed again I would most likely be leaving the hospital on Monday, unless there was some drastic turn of events.

I guess my highlight of weekend, other than the fact I was probably going to be able to get out of the hospital the next day, came when Linda thought I might not be enjoying some of the pureed food I was being served, and she thought I would enjoy some ripe, tasty bananas. The only problem was they weren't the yellow things we normal people find in the supermarket. She thought I would enjoy some bananas in the form of baby food; boy, was she wrong. I do think Gerber's and Temple must share recipes on some of the concoctions they try to pass off as food. I thanked her for her kindness and for being so thoughtful and told her she really shouldn't have, and I did mean she shouldn't have brought me that little treat. By the way, she did get the remaining containers of bananas returned to her in her Christmas stocking. Somehow I don't think I have seen the last of those bananas!

Like I said early on, having family is really great for the spirit when you are confined to the hospital.

Monday morning, September 30, 2013, arrived with much anticipation from me. Yes, the day still started early with the same routine: up at 6:00 a.m., vitals taken, out of bed, bathed, meds administered, ready for breakfast and in my chair just waiting to be discharged. Once again it seemed like I was back in the Army… hurry up and wait. I had to wait for the doctors to make their rounds and give their final thumbs up and have the transplant nurse come in and make certain I/we understood my discharge instructions. The doctors were late making their rounds, and the nurse was even later.

During my stay at Temple as a patient and especially while I was waiting to be discharged, I had a lot of time to think and reflect over the years since I had been diagnosed with IPF. I realized my being diagnosed with IPF changed my life and probably Karen's life entirely. Physically my pace had slowed dramatically; I did not like to exercise nor could I, and I avoided hills and stairs the best I could. I couldn't do the things I wanted to do; following the activities of our grandkids became a chore, and I couldn't do any traveling with Karen. Now since the transplant, I have hopes that after becoming stronger and as my recovery progresses, I will be able to do all of those things, I had not been able to do and more.

I have nothing but praise and good things to say about all the staff, nurses, doctors, and especially the surgeons while I was a patient here at Temple. I was treated like a person and not as an object. So far, our choice of going to Temple had been nothing but a positive experience. Any bumps in the road at Temple had been minor, but nothing to make me regret the choice we made.

While transplantation can greatly improve the quality of my life, it also demands much of me. I need to become and remain an active participant in preserving my health.

The average length of stay in the Intensive Care Unit is normally three to seven days; I was only there for one day before they moved me to the hospital side. The expected stay in the hospital is normally three to five weeks; I was out of the hospital in a total of eight days. Oh well, back to reality now.

The doctors came, and they were happy and said I could leave the hospital. Now I had to wait for Karen Steinke, the pulmonary transplant nurse, to come in and give us the discharge instructions. About noon she finally came in, and the second part of the discharge session began. I had forgotten she had been in a couple of days earlier to start these sessions. Boy, it is amazing what drugs will do your mind and memory, at least that is what I will blame it on. I am really thankful Karen was with me again to help me through these discharge instructions. I think I remember telling Karen S. she would do better if she would direct her conversation to my Karen since I had been known to doze off quite frequently during my stay at the hospital.

The discharge sessions were quite intensive. They went over everything I could and could not do. They did medication teaching, immunosuppression precautions, home monitoring, nutrition, health maintenance, daily activity, and outpatient follow-up.

Probably in my mind the medication training was the most important to me. Transplantation has become so successful in recent years in large part due to the development of new drugs, which prevent rejection of donated organs. These drugs inhibit the body's immune system from identifying the new organ as foreign. It will be necessary for me to take some of this medication for the rest of my life. A successful transplant could be undermined very quickly by my failure to take my medications appropriately and responsibly. We went over each medication, how often it was to be taken, and why I was taking it. All in all, the number of medications I will be required to take is relatively small, compared to medications others may be taking. When I left the hospital that day, my med list included the following medications: Cellcept (anti-rejection), Prograf (anti-rejection), Prednisone (anti-rejection), Bactrim DS (anti-viral), VFend (anti-fungal), Prilosec (stomach), Pravastatin (cholesterol), Lasix (diuretic), and Magnesium 64 (supplement). These medications will be adjusted periodically; some will go away and be replaced by others, some I will stop taking altogether, and others I will be taking for the rest of my life.

I was not allowed to drive for eight weeks. I didn't think I was going to like that, but it turned out okay. To this day, I still enjoy riding in the car and being able to look around. There is just so much you miss when you drive. I couldn't sit in the front seat of a car, but riding in a truck was okay. The reason for this is the fact you cannot turn the airbag off in a car like you can in a truck. The problem was not sitting in the front seat, but rather being exposed to the chemicals in an airbag in the unlikely event it would deploy. I couldn't clean the litter box or brush the cats - no exposure to indoor construction. The indoor construction might be a problem since they were laying hardwood flooring as we were having our discharge session; more on this later. I couldn't have birds or lizards as pets; I didn't see that happening anyway, and I definitely wasn't allowed to get any new pets. And of course I was pretty much banned from having alcohol, except on my two birthdays: my actual birthday and the date of my transplant. This has not been a problem, and quite honestly at this point I am not sure I will even have a drink when I am allowed.

Of course they stressed the importance of keeping all scheduled appointments at the outpatient clinic. In fact, my first appointment was scheduled for Thursday, October 4. Follow-up care initially involves returning to the outpatient clinic once a week for the first month after leaving the hospital. At this time a series of tests, including blood tests, were conducted to closely monitor my progress. This is a period when medications are adjusted. After this initial period of relatively intensive follow-up, I would be seen periodically as determined by my recovery.

Life After Transplant
(09/30/2013 and beyond)

The moment we had been waiting for had arrived: the nurse came and took the remaining IV port out of my arm, signed a couple of more papers, and we were free to go. The nurse wanted to call for a wheelchair to take me to the exit, but I would have none of that. I wanted to walk out of the hospital, just as I had walked in eight days earlier. Although it sounded like a good idea at the time, I apparently had forgotten how far the exit was. It certainly was farther than I had remembered. I guess the reward for my walking out of the hospital was the bench outside the exit where I could bask in the sun for a few minutes while I waited for my best friend and chauffer for the next eight weeks to come and pick me up to take us to the next stop on our journey with my lung transplant.

Sitting in the sun waiting for Karen to get the car felt so great, another experience I had taken for granted during my past 64 years. Unless you have experienced being confined, you might not understand the feelings I was having at this time.

My car and driver arrived, I wanted to get in the front seat with the driver, but she boldly pointed to the back seat and said if I was going to ride with her, my new seat, at least for the immediate future, was going to be in the back. I was going to be a real backseat driver!

We were going to be staying at the GOLF House for a couple of days for two reasons: one, we had my first weekly doctor's appointment in a couple of days and, two, our home was not quite clean enough for me to return to. I mentioned earlier that while I was in the hospital we had hardwood flooring put down in our home, and it was still quite dusty and not a suitable place for someone who had just had a lung transplant. Our cleaning crew, all family members, promised it would be ready in a day or two. This was a heck of a way to get our house cleaned.

The ride to Center City Philly was uneventful other than the fact the streets really, really, really needed to be repaved. I think we hit every hole or bump in the road, and my body felt every one of them, and let me tell you, my left side let me know it was not a happy camper. Ouch!

We did spend a few days at the GOLF House after I was discharged from the hospital. I wasn't completely happy about the extended stay in Philadelphia, but I understood.

Taking a shower and shaving for the first time in eight days was first on my agenda. The shower was better than I anticipated; changing into clean clothes would have been another Kodak moment if someone had been there with a camera, but fortunately no one was. The clothes brought from home didn't fit quite as snugly as they did before the transplant. I put my pants on, put a belt on, and they immediately dropped to the floor. Karen and I had a good laugh about this. Keep in mind I had lost about 40 pounds since I entered the hospital.

Keeping with the thought of exercise and staying healthy, I thought I had enough strength and energy to go for a short walk around the GOLF House. I quickly found out that was not going to be the case, I tired quickly, and soon I had to find a place to rest. The doctors at the hospital had told me my body would let me know if I was overdoing anything, and I guess this short walk was a bit too much for me to handle.

After my first of many post-transplant doctor's appointments, we headed west on the turnpike toward Harrisburg. It sure seemed funny sitting in the backseat of a car for such a long period of time, but I had eight weeks to get used to it. Returning home was a great feeling; when I had left almost two weeks earlier, I wasn't sure I would ever return.

Our youngest daughter Megan came in from Wisconsin to visit and help out for a few days. It was good to see her, and it alleviated quite a few questions she had about me and my recovery. It was good to visit with her, but it also provided Karen a little relief, and she was able to get away for a couple of hours to decompress.

That first doctor's appointment and almost every appointment since have been positive with no real issues uncovered. Like I said, there were a couple of bumps along the way, but I managed to come through them with minimal discomforts. One biopsy a couple of weeks after my release showed a minor rejection. A tweak of the Prednisone I was taking and I was on the road to getting back to my new normal, whatever that is.

Careful, comprehensive post-surgical monitoring allows the transplant team to constantly evaluate whether my body is accepting the new lung. This includes regular lung X-rays, bronchoscopies, and periodic biopsies. Biopsies are performed through a bronchoscope inserted into the airway and passing a delicate scissor device through the airway branches and into the lung under X-ray (fluoroscopy) guidance. Several small pieces of the lung are removed for microscopic examination.

The biopsy is important: if the doctors see evidence of immune injury to the lung (infiltration of cells called "lymphocytes"), then additional therapy may be prescribed to reverse this acute rejection process. Most transplant patients have four and sometimes five biopsies in the first year. I just had my second one on September 10, 2014.

For the first month I had appointments every week. After a while, the appointments were moved to every two weeks, and then it became a monthly appointment. Right now my appointments are every three months.

My doctors will say my recovery has been remarkable; other than the first and only bout of rejection I have recovered quite well. Up until a couple of months ago I was having blood work done weekly, and then it was changed to monthly. Having blood work done is one of the ways the medical staff control the medicines I am taking and also check for signs of rejection. Compared to others, a year out I am only taking five prescribed medicines daily; some patients are taking three or four times as many as I am.

Once friends found out I was home, I thought we may need to put in a revolving door on the front of the house. People wanted to visit and bring food for us. It was great to see family and friends, but to be honest, it was best Karen limited visiting hours because it sure tired me out. Don't get me wrong: I wanted to visit with people, but a couple of times I found myself taking a nap while friends were here.

During the month of October, I wanted to start walking on a regular basis so I could build up my strength and stamina. Karen took me over to the mall so we could walk indoors and out of the weather. I found out quickly it is going to take a while before I could walk any distance.

I did have to return during the first month to see my favorite speech therapist; she wasn't exactly convinced I was swallowing properly. I needed two additional appointments with her and two barium swallow tests were needed before she was satisfied I could swallow properly and would release me. I don't think either of us was particularly thrilled at these appointments. I guess you could say we had a love-hate relationship, but in a good way. I know she was doing her job and she was looking out for my best interests. The speech therapist finally was satisfied enough with my swallow tests and she released me a week or so prior to Thanksgiving. It was probably good she was satisfied with my test results because I was not going to miss Thanksgiving dinner.

Thanksgiving was extra special for Karen and me this year, especially me; we had a lot to be thankful for. We had a lot of people we needed to thank so far on this journey, and we weren't sure how we could manage that. We usually prepare the annual Thanksgiving meal at our house, but quite honestly I don't believe either of us was up to the preparation this year. Even if we were, I think all the activity would have been too much for me. We decided this year we would take our family out for dinner. This was our small way of starting to say thank you to a lot of people.

Here we were, heading toward winter and into the Christmas season; my recovery continued to be amazing. Other than needing to have blood drawn in Harrisburg, I did not have any appointments. Any adjustments needed to my medications were done over the phone. The medical staff at Temple continued to be impressed by my recovery. I did not have an appointment with them until the beginning of January 2014.

2014... A new year was upon us, and I was three plus months post-transplant. We were invited to spend New Year's at the beach. Although I felt pretty good, I was not sure this would be a good idea, so we declined, and Karen and I brought in the New Year as we normally do: we try to stay awake, wake up to watch the ball in Times Square drop, wish each other a Happy New Year, wait for the kids to call, and then go to bed. As usual we had pork and sauerkraut for dinner on New Year's Day; after all, isn't that supposed to bring us luck for the rest of year?

Winter arrived here, and I am certain you have heard of "the battle of the sexes"; here at the Carns household we were having "the battle of the thermostat"! Since my transplant in September, it's been apparent to me and others that I have trouble getting warm. I can often be found wearing a sweatshirt on days where others might be out sweating their a$$'s off. With that being said, maybe you can figure out what might be coming next. You got it... here it was the middle of January, and I am guessing we might not have seen the coldest weather yet, and I can't get warm. Even if I have the heat in the house cranked up to 74 degrees, wore a flannel shirt, sweater, sweatshirt and sat in front of the fireplace wrapped up in a blanket, I'm still cold. I guess some day this too will pass. Heck, if I was cold then, what is it going to be like when the air conditioner is turned on this summer?

We did go to TUH for my scheduled appointment on January 8, and we did not come home disappointed. Everything was great, and nothing new was uncovered. They still were tinkering with my medications to get all my levels where they were supposed to be. My next appointment was scheduled for late March, not bad for someone who had had a lung transplant three months earlier.

Remember I wrote previously about asking the doctors to get their a$$ in gear and find lungs for me because we wanted to go to Alaska in 2014? Well, we asked if they thought it would be possible for us to start making arrangements. To our surprise, they had no objections; the only thing that was suggested was we made certain we had travel insurance just in case something came up and we had to cancel our trip.

Toward the end of the month, the weather turned quite wintery in Harrisburg. The snow and sleet came with a vengeance. Karen learned to use the snow blower in a hurry. While she did her share of snow blowing, the neighbors were often there to help out. Like I said earlier, the people we needed to thank are too numerous to mention. I really felt bad I couldn't help out with the snow shoveling, but I understand why. I must admit, Karen sometimes came in from the outside covered from head to foot in snow. Quite frankly, I think she enjoyed being out in the weather.

February starts the same way January ended: cold and snowy. I must admit when I did go out and help a little bit with the snow I wasn't much help, but I did help a little. In the grand scheme of things, it was darn little.

Karen did remark she "**mastered**" the use of the snow blower, but I told her she didn't perfect it. For some reason she took offense to my observation and told me the job of clearing the driveway and sidewalks would be my job this year. I guess I am still a slow learner and don't know when to keep my mouth shut. I must say Karen continues to go above and beyond when called upon to come out of her comfort zone.

The progress of my recovery still was going quite smoothly. Other than a bout of the flu, (so much for flu shots) I continued on what we considered a remarkable recovery. I did start pulmonary rehab this month. I went and worked out on the machines and walked on the treadmill at my own pace. At times this seemed to annoy the people who were monitoring my recovery. When I left the hospital, the doctors told me I really had no restrictions, and I could do what my body would allow. If I would overdo something, my body would let me know in no uncertain terms.

I started writing a letter of thanks to my donor family; in fact, I had started this letter many times over the previous several months, and believe me, the words just don't flow as easily as one would think. It is difficult to come up with words to express one's thanks and gratitude for the gift I received on September 22, 2013. Instead of trying to put into words the difficulty I had, it will be so much easier if I just include a copy of this in my journal. Since I was not to have any direct contact with the donor family, I had to send this through the Gift of Life Donor Program, who in turn forwarded it to the donor family.

I wrote the following letter to say thank you for allowing his organs to be donated so others would have a chance at living. I don't know if I will ever hear from this family, but I would certainly hope that I will have an opportunity to meet them and to thank them in person for this unselfish act.

February 18, 2014

Dear Donor Family:

My name is Jim, and I am the 64-year-old retired male who received the precious gift from your loved one. I know there are no words that can truly express my feelings for your family; it takes a special kind of person to make such a sacrifice in their time of grief and need. I would like you to know your loved one and your families are in my thoughts and prayers every day. I know I will never be able to thank you enough for giving me a second chance at life.

In 2010 I was diagnosed with pulmonary fibrosis and on September 22, 2013 I received the left lung from your loved one. You, he/she and your loved ones left lung quite possibly saved my life. I promise I will take care of this special gift I received. Each night before I go to sleep and each morning before I get out of bed I take a moment to reflect on this gift steadily pumping life sustaining oxygen through my body. It is alive and healthy and has created in me a new appreciation for life.

I thought you might like to know the doctors say everything is progressing extremely well. I have had no major signs of rejection and the left lung is functioning extremely well. It has been almost five months since the operation at the time I am writing this letter. I would have written sooner, but I wanted to make sure everything was working out so I could show you what has been accomplished by your family's decision to donate.

I am aware that lung is not mine. It belonged to the kind of person all of us should want to be. Maybe it is my imagination but since receiving my new lung, I feel a peace I haven't felt before.

I appreciate the simple things now, much more than before. I look forward every morning to seeing my loving wife and caregiver, Karen. Each day gives me a new thrill because each day is a gift from you and from God.

My hope is one day we will meet so I can personally say thank you to you and your family. When that does happen, I will likely be at a loss for words; I would like to thank you personally. You gave me life, you gave me peace and you gave me a profound sense of gratitude and understanding. I am a new person and I hope in your grief it helps to know a part of your loved one is alive and with his help I am trying to live my life in a way that would make you proud.

My wife and I would also like to say how sorry we are for your loss. It is nice to know there are such special people in this world who care about other people so much.

Saying thank you just doesn't seem like enough when what somebody does is basically save your life. I sincerely hope life treats your family to nothing but happiness and prosperity. If there is anything you would like to know about or from me, please feel free to contact me.

Again, I just want to say thank from the bottom of my heart.

Jim

I started pulmonary rehab again, and while I was there continuing my recovery, I met several people who had been diagnosed with IPF and invited each one of them to come to our support group meetings at the Hershey Medical Center. I am convinced that participating in a support group is beneficial to not only the patient, but also the caregiver. More on support groups later.

Remember when I was going through the evaluation process they told me I had an abscessed tooth? Well, lo and behold, that very same tooth that wasn't abscessed then started to give me trouble. I went to the dentist, and he suggested I either go and have another root canal done or have it pulled. I reluctantly chose to have it pulled. Another first in my book: 64 years old and I had my first tooth pulled.

March came in sort of like a lamb; the snow and sleet had subsided, but now it had started to rain. Oh well, at least we don't have to shovel it, or I should say, Karen doesn't have to shovel it!

We were invited to attend a reception for the GOLF House. It just so happens it was the evening prior to my appointment at Temple, so we were able to attend. It was nice to be able to talk not only to those who have received transplants, but also to hear from family members who were involved directly with the organ donation process.

The appointment on March 20 was uneventful; my recovery continues to go forward without any major issues. My PFTs show my lung capacity continues to increase with each test I do. The doctors still aren't happy with my medications, and they are still trying to get them leveled out; I think they are getting closer.

April is here already, and it is time to get ready for the Easter Bunny. Signs of spring are popping up everywhere. Some flowers are starting to come out, and the grass is getting green and will soon need to be mowed. One of my goals for this year is to mow my own grass. Our grandson does a good job, but he doesn't have it perfected yet. ☺ We had Easter dinner here at the house, and everyone helped out by preparing a portion of the meal. Recovery still seems to be progressing without problems, other than the doctors are still tweaking my medications.

May is here, and I will soon be celebrating my eight-month anniversary. Another goal for 2014 was to play golf again, so since I haven't played for quite some time, Karen got me golf lessons for Christmas, and heaven knows I would need them. Just like anything else I want to do, I called Temple and asked if swinging a golf club would be a problem. There was dead silence on the other end of the phone when I asked! The response other than the silence and a chuckle and mild laughter was, "Probably not going to happen." Since my side is still achy, they said if I golf, I will probably just aggravate those muscles more. Another good idea I had, but I guess I will need to put golfing on hold for a little while longer.

I had an appointment with Dr. Meshkov, the cardiologist, on May 27. He did another EKG, and nothing unexpected was found. The heart is still strong.

We participated in the Highmark Walk for a Healthy Community on the 17th. We walked in support of our IPF Support Group, which is named Sweet Lungs of Mine and in honor of my donor. Karen and I raised almost $3,000, which will go toward research to help find a cure for IPF. It was a beautiful day, and we had no problem finishing the 5K course. If I had not received my new lung, I wonder if I would have been able to participate this year. My guess is I would have been sitting on the sidelines cheering our team on.

We finally attended one of Temple's IPF support group meetings. This had been strongly suggested to us since we started going to Temple. We attended not because it had been strongly suggested, but rather the topic was one we thought would benefit us. The topic was traveling after transplant. Since we had the trip to Alaska planned, we thought it would be worthwhile

Still feeling good, still doing monthly blood tests, and still adjusting my medications, but compared to a year ago, there is no comparison as to how I feel.

June is here. I had to call Temple to see if it is okay for me to go to Hershey Park with two of our grandkids. I told them it is my goal to ride all of the roller coasters if possible. The doctors had no problem, and their only advice was to make sure I don't throw up and to remember to take my medicine. I told them it was not my intention to get sick, but if I did, they would be one of the first ones to know. I had a great day, rode most of the coasters, some of them multiple times. I will admit I did sleep quite well that night because it did tire me out.

Karen went to visit a friend near Atlantic City for a couple of days, and I got to stay by myself. This is the first time she had gone somewhere and didn't have anybody check on me. I guess I am back to being a big boy now and can stay **all** by myself.

We had my final pre-Alaskan doctor's visit and they gave me their blessing to go and enjoy. You don't know what that meant to us. This is the trip I jokingly suggested to the doctor we wanted to take if I had the transplant. I don't know if Dr. Cordova was listening or not, but I am sure God was!

36

Another good appointment; we like those kind if appointments, and I don't need to go back until the end of September, which will be for my one year anniversary checkup.

I got a phone call from our friend Bill and he told me he just got the word he has been listed. To me that was great news. He was bummed because his LAS was low, and he says with a number as low as his, it would be a long time until he would get his transplant. I reminded him my number was also low, and I was only listed for about three months before I got my call. Little did he know or realize two days later, on June 28, he would get his call his gift was ready, and he would be the recipient of a double lung transplant. We talked with his wife after his surgery, and she told us all was going as well as expected. What great news that was for us to start our Alaskan vacation.

July came, and Alaska, here we come. The meds are all counted out, and extra pills are also counted. I am not certain why I had to pack a week's worth of extra pills because I had no plans to extend this trip The bottom line was we had a great trip, and we were grateful. It was important to me just to be able to spend those two weeks with Karen. I wore my mask on each of our flights, and that sure does get the stares from people, and not just the little ones. At first that was a little uncomfortable, but I kept reminding myself I was not protecting them from me, but rather I was protecting myself from them.

When we were in Fairbanks I met a lady who was carrying an oxygen tank, and I struck up a conversation with her, and we shared our stories. She tells me she has IPF, and this trip was on her bucket list and will probably be her last trip anywhere. She told me she does not qualify for transplant at Duke University and is currently looking at other options she might have. It's funny to me because prior to my being diagnosed with IPF; I probably would not have gone up to a stranger and started a conversation about health issues, now it is different. I have no problem starting a conversation, especially if I think he or she might be fighting this terrible disease. I don't offer solutions; I might have opinions, but I often find just listening is helpful.

All of the overland bus travel we were doing made me quite tired, and to be honest, most days I was glad to see our hotel room at the end of the day. The tour people sure kept us moving, but that was what we signed up to do.

37

I was looking forward to the cruise portion of our trip because I thought the pace might slow down and we/I could relax a bit. WRONG. This was just a different kind of activity. We also had a great time. Karen decides to add a little adventure to the trip; she needs to catch a cold. It was bad enough she caught a cold, but she decides she needs to share it with me. I got sick, and that really slowed me down for a few days. She says I would have caught it anyway, but I think she just wanted to share. You all know that is just the kind of person she is.

All in all, this was a great trip. We saw many different things, met a lot of great people, and most of all I spent two weeks with my favorite person. A year ago we had doubts I would have been able to do this trip. In fact, there was probably doubt I would ever be able to do any trip, but with God's help, modern medical technology, and the support of family and friends, it was possible.

In hindsight, which is better than no sight at all, it was probably a bit soon for me to take off on a two-week vacation anywhere, but we did it, and it was a great experience I wouldn't change for anything. Well, I could have done without the cold I brought home with me ….

No trips to Philadelphia this month as long as I have no problems. I didn't have to go east on the turnpike. Yea………..

August is here, and I feel pretty good except I can't shake this cold or whatever it is I have, and I have been tiring out extremely quickly. I will admit I don't have the energy I had four or five months ago. They had me do additional blood tests, which showed my white blood count was extremely low. We need to get it back to an acceptable range. Once again they tell me my meds will probably be changing. They wanted to know if I could give myself injections in the abdomen if needed; not a thought I was going to relish, but you do what you have to do. To make a long story short, the doctors change my medication, and decided against my using a needle. I thought that was a good decision on their part, at least I initially thought it was a good decision. Temple called in a prescription, and the CVS pharmacy gave me a courtesy call to tell me not only was my prescription ready for pickup, but my co-pay would be in excess of $800; I suggested they not fill this prescription at the present time. It seems I have fallen into the proverbial

38

donut hole you often hear about; another long story made short is I went to the VA and got my drug for $24. As consumers we wonder: why the difference in the cost of drugs?

Although I had been back to Temple quite a few times since my discharge, this has been my first time I had the opportunity to visit someone. It was sort of a surreal experience getting off of the elevator on the sixth floor; the room I was in, even though nobody was in it, looked just like I remembered. This is the first time I have been back on the sixth floor since I was discharged. When I was discharged in September, the nurses told me they didn't want to see me back on the floor unless it was to visit.

I still wasn't able to shake the remnants of my cold, and although I have been remaining active, I have been tiring quite quickly and often found myself napping more often. Although I wasn't scheduled to go back to Temple until late September, we wanted to get this checked out earlier, rather than later. This is the first time since the transplant I couldn't wait until my next scheduled appointment. Dr. Cordova was out of the office, so I was able to get an appointment with Dr. Criner. Dr. Criner is another doctor at Temple who is a leading doctor in this field. Health wise, except for the cold, they were satisfied there was nothing seriously wrong with me, gave me another prescription to knock out this cold and suggested I make an appointment for a sleep study to see if that might be a cause of my being tired all the time.

Last winter I was sort of looking forward to the "warmth" of the summer months. I must admit, it was not quite what I had expected. Remember how I said I had difficulty getting warm when it was cold outside? Well, believe it or not, while everyone was hot and sweaty and enjoying the summer months, I was still the one sitting around wearing the sweatshirt. When Karen cranked (whatever the appropriate word is) the air conditioner up or down, I was the one banished to the front or back porch to sit in the sun to get warm. Once again, I was the one wearing the sweatshirt in 95-degree weather, and I was the one causing people to stare and wonder: what is wrong with the man in the sweatshirt?

All in all, I must say dealing with staying warm sure as heck beats the alternative for me.

September is here, and I am approaching my one-year anniversary, and this is going to be a busy month. Karen wanted to arrange a birthday party of sorts to be celebrated on the 22nd. Although it was a great idea and heaven knows I/we have a lot to celebrate, I didn't want to have a party. There were a couple of reasons why I was opposed. First, in order to have a real celebration, I would want to invite everybody who was a part of this journey we have been on. While this number would have been many, I am sure I would have left somebody out, and I didn't want that to happen. Second, I didn't want to celebrate the gift I received while I knew there was another family somewhere probably still mourning the loss of a loved one.

I had to go to Temple to have some tests done as part of my "First Anniversary" check-up. I had blood tests, chest X-rays, a CT scan, and the pulmonary function tests. The following day I was supposed to be there at 7:00 a.m. for a 7:30 bronchoscopy/biopsy; they called and changed the time to be there to 9:00 a.m. for the 9:30 procedure. Not a problem; that just meant an extra hour of sleep for us. We got there on time and went to get ready and went back to the waiting area and waited and waited and waited.... Well, you get the idea. At 2:45 p.m. they wheeled me into the procedure room. It was late until we got home that evening. I needed to have these tests done for my appointment at the end of the month, and we would go over the results at that time. We assume if anything showed up on these tests that need to be addressed prior to my appointment, they will call us.

We traveled to Pittsburgh to attend the annual Pulmonary Fibrosis Advocacy Event that is held each year. Leading doctors and researchers come together to talk about what is happening with IPF. This was the same conference we attended in 2011 when we were just beginning our journey. We attended this conference when it was held in Harrisburg; this was our first real contact with patients, caregivers, the medical staffs and researchers looking for a cure for this disease. Karen and I both thought this was a worthwhile event and recommend it to anyone suffering from IPF. A lot of information was shared, and it gave us the opportunity to talk with others who were on this journey with IPF.

Well, the big day is here: I made it a year with the gift I received from an unknown 36-year-old man. To his family I owe much gratitude for allowing his organs to be used to help others. This 36- year-old man gave me a gift so

I might be able to have some sort of a normal life. I know for certain he did not leave home that day saying, "I am going to die today, and I want to give Jim Carns my left lung." Let's face it; I am quite aware of how this process works: someone's life ends, probably too soon, and someone else gets a chance to live on. I am very blessed to have received this gift. I feel confident I might not have been the sickest person on the transplant list, but all the stars aligned properly and I was the perfect match for this special gift. Don't get me wrong, this was bound to happen, but I believe Karen and I both thought it would be later rather than sooner. At some point I hope and pray I will have the opportunity to meet his family and personally thank them for making the decision to donate life and let them see their loved one lives on through me.

For the most part I feel great; compared to last year, there really is no comparison. I can do many more things that were far out of my reach prior to my transplant. In the past year I have been able to travel, enjoy the grandkids and their activities, mow my own grass, go to the park, spend time at the beach, walk more than short distances, exercise, help around the house more, and I don't need oxygen.

We went down to Temple for my checkup, and as expected, no real issues were brought up. We reviewed the tests, and they were all positive, nothing out of the ordinary to report, so all in all it was a good checkup. The only downside to this appointment was when Dr. Cordova asked if I had had the sleep test done yet. I told him it was scheduled for next month and I wasn't thrilled about participating in this test. I told him I had done this test before. We talked about my reasoning, and he said if I didn't want to, I didn't have to. Then he asked me when I had had this test done. I told him it had probably been about 15 years or so since I had done the sleep study. That apparently was not the correct answer. He looked at us and said I should do the study and then we would talk about the results at my next appointment. I don't go back for my next appointment until January 2015.

October is here already, and I am starting the next year of my journey with IPF. I say continue my journey because I had a single lung transplant, my native lung remains in my body and still is fibrotic, and is functioning at a greatly reduced capacity.

It is now time to, as they say, "Pay it Forward" for what we have received while guests at the GOLF House in Philadelphia. Karen and I decided we would prepare a home-cooked meal for the guests on October 2. With the help of our family, we did steaks on the grill, baked potatoes, baked beans, salad, and an assortment of desserts. This meal was something other than chicken or pasta dishes, which is what they get plenty of. We understand people and organizations prepare those types of meals because of the ease of preparation. We had fun preparing the meal and talking with the people who were there for various reasons. Some were there for appointments, and some were there because they had a loved one in one of the area transplant hospitals. After all, it wasn't long ago Karen and I were the ones on the receiving end of the meals. It was a great feeling to be able to give back. Everybody enjoyed this meal and the effort we made to make their day a little brighter.

Our IPF Group manned a table at a local fire house near our home. Our goal was to help make the public aware of what pulmonary fibrosis is and how it affects people from all walks of life.

In early October we participated in the local Crop Walk. On the surface there is nothing special about this: it is something millions of others have done before me, but for me it was something special. You see, in the past three or four years, I was not able to complete this 5K course for various reasons related to my IPF and lung transplant. Even though this was only 3.2 miles, in the past, because of my IPF, I needed oxygen, became short of breath, or just became too tired to finish. This year was different. Not only was I able to complete the course, but I was able to walk it at a fairly fast pace, didn't really become short of breath, and really didn't become too tired to finish. For me this was a major accomplishment I can cross off my list. Like I said, for most people this is no big deal, but for me it certainly was.

Remember a while back I told you Dr. Cordova and Dr. Criner thought it would be a good idea if I had a sleep apnea test to rule out apnea as the reason I was becoming tired so frequently? Well, that day, or should I say night, arrived. I went to my appointment and tried to fall asleep. Do you realize how difficult it is to fall asleep with sensors and wires protruding from various areas of your body? I eventually fell asleep, and I thought I slept rather soundly. I did wake myself three times by my count because of my arm and shoulder being uncomfortable and rolled over and went to sleep again. Did I wake up other times because of this? Maybe, but I am certain I didn't wake up gasping for breath because I couldn't breathe. Did I snore? Who knows? I didn't hear it if I did snore, and nobody was pounding on the wall to tell me to knock it off.

I could go on and on about this sleep apnea test, but I will stop right now before I start to sound "whiny". Does this sound to you like I might have a little bit of an attitude? If you guessed yes from reading this journal, you would be absolutely correct. Probably this ranks right up there with the speech therapist and her swallowing tests. In fact, my attitude is worse than it was 12 or 13 months ago when I was on that pureed diet.

I received a call from our friend Bill, who had the double lung transplant back in June, asking if Karen and I would like to join him and his wife to be interviewed by one of the local Upper Dauphin County newspapers. He asked if we wanted to help get the word out about IPF since it is a disease most people have never heard of. We jumped at this opportunity and even suggested he might want to include another one of our friends so he could provide another perspective about this disease.

We were interviewed by a reporter from the *Upper Dauphin Sentinel*. All in all, I thought it was a couple of hours well spent telling our stories with the hope we will be able to make more people aware of this deadly disease. I can't wait to see when this article goes to press and what the final article will look like. We asked Bill and his wife to get us a couple of copies when it hits the newsstand. This article appears starting on the next page.

We received the quarterly newsletter from GOLF House and saw Karen and I made the front cover of the newsletter. Our smiling faces were right in the center. A couple of months ago we were interviewed by a Philadelphia writer for an article to be used for GOLF House annual fundraising edition. We had no problem doing this interview because we do support this organization 100% and, like we said in the article, "We fell in love with this place."

I was asked to participate in a research project at the Hershey Medical Center. They asked if I would be interested in participating as a patient partner. As a patient partner, I will help the PaTH team understand what research questions matter most to patients with IPF, help make sure the rights and privacy of patients are protected, and help design studies that are real and meaningful to patients. I will be working mainly with IPF patients although there will be two other groups participating: one is on obesity and the other has to do with atrial fibrillation (AF).

I do know that on this project I will have the opportunity to work with Dr. Kevin Gibson from UPMC, Dr. Francis Cordova from TUH, and Kathy Lindell from UPMC as well as Dr. Rebecca Bascom from Penn State Hershey.

I think it is worth noting at this time an update on the Pirfenidone study I participated in prior to my transplant. On October 15, 2014, the U.S. Food & Drug administration approved the use of Pirfenidone, now called Esbriet for the treatment of idiopathic pulmonary fibrosis here in the United States. It feels pretty darn good being a part of history in the making. OFEV was also approved at this time.

November is here, and I am starting the 14th month since my transplant, and I have plenty to be thankful for during this upcoming holiday season.

Well, it didn't take long for the "brain trust" in Philadelphia to call and suggest strongly I should continue with getting fitted for a CPAP mask. They told me I have a tendency to stop breathing for short periods of time. I may not like the idea, and I might disagree I need the CPAP machine, but I promised a lot of people I would do whatever the doctors tell me to do to keep the "gift" I received healthy. I took the first available appointment the sleep center had, so I could return for part two of the sleep study early in December. Hey, it's not my fault I couldn't get in sooner!

Bill called and said our interview was in the November 13, 2014, edition of the *Upper Dauphin Sentinel*. I immediately went online, and the following is what was written. I must say this article was pretty much what we said during the interview. It didn't take long for us to send copies to family and friends.

New lungs bring new life

Area man diagnosed with rare disease,

Idiopathic pulmonary fibrosis, needed transplant

Story and [sic] by Shirley Brosius

Through the years, Bill Mattern of Washington Twp. loved his work. Whether maintaining storage units or a mobile home park, working in his construction business or more recently working at Koppy's Propane, he was on the go. He and his wife Ellen wintered in Florida and enjoyed travel.

All that changed in 2006. Mattern had always run up the sloped driveway from his home to his shop, but suddenly exertion tired him. He became short of breath climbing ladders. And he developed a dry, hacking cough.

"I usually was a person who didn't let things like that get to me too much," he said.

But Mattern was forced to seek medical treatment, and in 2008, doctors diagnosed idiopathic pulmonary fibrosis (IPF), a terminal condition in which lung tissue becomes scarred and hardens and can no longer process the exchange of blood oxygen. Mattern was 58 at the time.

The disease slowly progressed, and on a trip west, while visiting the Grand Canyon in 2009, it became evident his condition had deteriorated.

"I had a problem with altitudes," he said, speaking through a mask he wears to protect himself when around visitors. "There were places we couldn't go because of the elevations."

In 2012, Mattern was evaluated and put on a waiting list for a single or double lung transplant. They would do either one as an organ or organs became available. By then he had been tethered to an oxygen tank for two years.

Then in January, while vacationing in Florida, Mattern found IPF severely affected his breathing. After returning to Pennsylvania, he was sent to pulmonary rehabilitation in

Harrisburg and at first felt stronger. He was able to walk the treadmill for 12 minutes at 1.5 miles per hour.

But during the third week of rehab, he walked for just three minutes and couldn't go on.

"I just (waved my hands) and said 'I got to stop,'" he said.

Tests showed he needed a lung transplant—immediately.

The next morning, June 28, he received a call from Temple University Hospital in Philadelphia telling him two lungs were available.

The surgery took eight hours, but Mattern emerged from it a changed man.

"Wow!" his wife Ellen exclaimed, throwing up her hands at the difference the surgery has made. "Unbelievable."

"Like flipping a light switch on me," Mattern added. "I can do anything I want to do now."

"We just have to hold him back," Ellen noted.

Claims 40,000 lives yearly. According to information published by the Coalition for Pulmonary Fibrosis, 40,000 people die from IPF annually, which is the same number who die of breast cancer.

The disease causes patients to gradually lose the ability to breathe as scar tissue (fibrosis) develops in the lungs. Half of the cases are misdiagnosed for a year or more.

Lung transplantation is currently the only treatment option, but 50 per cent of patients on a transplant list will die before they can receive a lung.

The Matterns have made new friends as they attend Hershey Idiopathic Pulmonary Fibrosis Support Group, a group of 20 to 30 patients and caregivers meets monthly.

One new friend is Jim Carns of Harrisburg, who received a single lung in September, 2013.

"This isn't a cure for us," he said. "It's going to give us an extension of life and hopefully a better quality of life than what we had. It sure beats carrying a tank of oxygen around."

Except for a high cholesterol reading, Carns had been a healthy man up until 2009, when, while hiking in Colorado, he realized he was still struggling to go up a hill while others were coming down.

He was diagnosed with IPF in 2010 and went for a second opinion in 2012.

"Early in 2013 we started the evaluation process, where we find out everything we didn't want to know about our body and more," he said, smiling.

On September 22, 2013, he got the call that a lung was available.

"(My wife) Karen picked it up and said 'This is the call you've been waiting for,'" Carns remembered.

They picked up his sister and by 11 a.m. he was on the operating table at Temple University Hospital in Philadelphia.

"You remember the day," he said. "It's like a birthday."

"Those lungs weren't meant for me." Park Barner of Harrisburg also attends the support group. His wife, Gail, also was diagnosed with IPF, but unfortunately did not survive.

Up until December, 2007, Gail Barner volunteered at a local food bank and at a library. She was active in her church, and the couple enjoyed walking in a state park close to their home.

But suddenly Gail became extremely tired, and a lung biopsy revealed IPF.

She was put on a transplant list in August 2011.

The Barners got a call that a lung was available for her during a snowstorm that October.

Neighbors shoveled their driveway so the couple could rush to the University of Pittsburgh Medical Center.

"They got her prepped and everything," Barner said, wiping his eyes. "I'm sitting there. The doctor comes in and said, 'Unfortunately, the donor's family changed their minds.' Whoaaa. What do you do now? We never thought that would happen."

They returned home physically, emotionally and mentally exhausted. For 26 months they waited for another call. It never came. Gail Barner died on December 18, 2013.

"She had a wonderful positive attitude," Ellen Mattern said. "When she didn't get the transplant, she said, 'Well, those lungs weren't meant for me."

Smaller "bucket lists." In September Park Barner attended the 2014 National PF Awareness Day in Washington D. C. in support of funding for greater research of the disease.

Two types of PF have been determined: idiopathic, which means "of unknown cause," and familial, which comes through a family's genes.

Mattern believes occupational hazards might have contributed to his illness. As a youth, he helped his father, who was an exterminator. Later in life he sprayed foam insulation.

Carns said his condition might have been caused by exposure to toxic substances in Vietnam, working in the steel industry, smoking or other factors: however, he stressed, there is no known cause for this disease.

Shortness of breath is one of the main symptoms of the disease. Mattern and Carns hold out their hands to show another: "clubbing" of the fingernails in which the ends of the nails hug the fingertip.

"Awareness is a really big thing," Karen Carns said. "If you learn what this is, you might (identify) symptoms early on before you're so sick."

According to Carns, finding out he had the disease threw him into denial.

"I was bitter," he said. "I worked my way through with the help of Karen and our minister. If you don't laugh you cry. That was my philosophy. It is what it is."

Both Mattern and Carns will take immuno suppressants for the rest of their lives along with a dozen or more other medications.

They appreciate each day of life.

"Our bucket lists have gotten a whole lot smaller," Carns said on his and Mattern's behalf. "Spending time with the family; I want to mow my own grass this year."

Mattern hopes to see his two grandchildren, now in college, graduate.

As he and Ellen recently drove along Route 6, in the northern tier he told her, "I honestly thought I wasn't going to be here to see the leaves turn color in fall. I didn't think I would see this."

According to the men, increased federal funding for research of PF is needed since the disease receives considerably less funding than other rare, deadly diseases that affect fewer people.

More Information For more information about the disease or to contribute to research funding or patient resources, visit the Coalition for Pulmonary Fibrosis website at www.coalitionforpf.org.

I haven't mentioned very much about support groups, so now might be a good time to do so. What is a support group, you may ask? Support groups are made up of people with common interests and experiences. People who have been through, or are going through, a similar circumstance can do more than sympathize with you — they can relate to what you are going through and keep you from feeling like you are alone.

We have been a part of the Penn State-Hershey support group since we became aware of their existence back in 2011. Since we were fairly new to IPF and how it affects not only the patient, but also the caregiver, we were always grasping for new information about this disease. We thought: what better place to go find out was going on than to meet with people who have been dealing with this same disease? We found out we could share our thoughts, express ourselves, vent when necessary, and no one sat in judgment. We met individuals who were just like us, just starting out on this journey, individuals who have been traveling this road for a while, people who have received the gift of life, and even individuals who had lost loved ones due to IPF.

We have a facilitator who is well versed on the disease and even two doctors who are doing research on lung disease. What better group of people to be associated with? We met people and have come to find out IPF does not discriminate; people from all walks of life are affected.

You might say we have become a close-knit family. We share our joys, celebrate our victories, and at times we come together to mourn our losses. All in all, we are there for each other.

Over the past three years, this IPF support group has become an important part of our lives. Although we only meet once a month, our meetings usually draw about 25-30 people, and usually we will find a newcomer has joined us. A newcomer is someone who is just starting out on his or her own journey and is seeking information about IPF and how it might affect him or her.

At each meeting we usually have a speaker who will talk on topics such as drug studies, pulmonary rehab, research, organ donations, exercise, or anything else that might be of interest to the group.

I know for me, part of my being listed for transplant included a strong suggestion I attend support group meetings held monthly at Temple, so that goes to show how important the hospitals think support groups are.

Here it is the day before the big feast we call Thanksgiving. This will be my second Thanksgiving since my transplant just over 14 months ago, and I for one have something to be thankful for when we gather around the table tomorrow.

Since I have something to be thankful for, Karen suggested now might be a good time to write another letter to my donor family. After all, if it weren't for the donor and his family, who knows how this journey of mine may have turned out. This letter was a little easier for me to write than the original one back in February. I attribute this to the fact I stressed and fretted through the first one to make certain my words were just right and came from my heart.

I wrote the following and forwarded it to the Gift of Life organization in Philadelphia, who in turn will forward it to my donor family. I keep hoping each time I go to our mailbox I will find a letter from my donors family. I have been told it is not unusual not to hear from them; sometimes it takes a while for the family to feel comfortable to send a response, and it is possible I will never get that letter that I keep hoping for.

November 27, 2014

Dear Donor Family,

Hi it's me again, Jim! It has been nine months since I last wrote and I continue to count my blessings each day.

I felt that this might be a good time for me to write and tell you how thankful I have been since I received the precious gift from your loved one. I continue to struggle finding the right words to say to you and your family. I would like you to know that your loved one and your family are in my thoughts and prayers every day. I know I will never be able to thank you enough for giving me a second chance at life.

The doctors continue to be quite pleased with my recovery and I feel stronger every day. I am not out running any distances yet, but I do try to keep active. Since the weather has changed, I have become a mall walker and walk on a regular basis and most days I walk 2 – 3 miles if not farther.

I had set a few goals for myself for this year; some which I thought would be doable for me. I wanted to mow my own lawn, which I did. My grandson was doing a great job, but there was something about the satisfaction of doing it on my own.

Since my wife had gotten me a gift certificate for a couple of golf lessons I wanted to do some golfing this year, but I quickly found out that I was not going to be able to accomplish that goal. When I tried to swing a golf club it became apparent that the muscles in my side have not healed enough to let me go out on the golf course to play at this time. Oh well I will try for next year.

Another goal was to be able to walk a mile in 15 minutes. Although I walk several miles a day, this goal has eluded me. It takes me about 16 or 17 minutes to do this so I still have some work to do.

I know those goals that I have set for myself seem small in comparison to what some others are facing; I keep remembering that fourteen months ago I would not have been able to do any of those goals or many other things that my wife and I have been able to do without the gift that I received from your loved one.

I continue hoping that one day, when the time is right, we will have the opportunity to meet so that I can personally say thank you to you and your family.

Your loved one continues to live through me and that with his help I am trying to live my life in a way that would make you proud.

I continue to hope that life treats your family to nothing but happiness and prosperity. If there is anything you would like to know about or from me, please feel free to contact me.

Again, I just want to say thank from the bottom of my heart.

Peace

[signature: Jim]

Well, here I am 14 months out, and I must say I feel, for the most part, pretty darn good. My only complaint is my achy side and still getting tired quickly. Other than that, considering how things could have turned out, life is good, and I am still much better off now than I was 14 months ago: I am not using oxygen, I get regular exercise, I walk two, three, or sometimes four miles a day, and do more physical things to help around the house. As we sit around the table this year, I/we have a lot to be thankful for this Thanksgiving Day.

December is here already, and it is hard to believe this year has passed by so quickly. It seems like it was just yesterday 2014 began, and now we will soon be celebrating the New Year.

The first Monday I provided the doctors with their monthly five vials of blood so they can check to make sure I am not showing signs of rejection and so they can make necessary adjustments to my medications if necessary. As I sit here and think about it, they haven't made any changes for a couple of months. To me this has been good news.

Temple Lung Center had a Christmas party for all lung transplant patients and Karen and I attended. I believe I heard someone say there were 32 patients who had undergone transplants in attendance. The transplant patients had received their gifts of life ranging from 15 years ago to a man who received a single lung back in September. It gave us the opportunity to see friends we have made while we have been on this journey. We had the opportunity to talk about our recoveries, both the positive things and things that haven't been so positive. It is always good to have the opportunity to be able to talk to others who have gone through lung transplantation. It was also good for Karen to be able to talk to other caregivers and also be able to compare notes on our transplants.

They announced so far in 2014 there have been 53 transplants through the month of November at Temple, and their goal for the entire year is 60.

The highlight of this day for me was meeting Dr. Shiosi, my transplant surgeon, and being able to talk to him while I was not under anesthesia or the influence of any drugs. I found it hard to comprehend he remembered who I was. I introduced myself as "September 22, 2013'", and while he didn't know my name, his response was, "Single left lung." This had really been the first time I could personally thank him for what a great job he and his team did over 14 months ago.

Christmas day is here, and as I look back, I still am reminded how blessed I have been for the last 14 months. Just like at Thanksgiving, I have so many things to be thankful for. Karen and I exchanged our gifts in the morning.

We will be celebrating the New Year in a few short days. We will be spending this holiday with some close friends at their beach house in Bethany Beach. Will I be making resolutions this year? Well, maybe a few. One will be to remain as healthy as possible and to take very good care of the gift I received. Another resolution will be to continue to honor the memory of the 36 year-old man who provided me with the gift of life. And lastly, I will pledge to continue to be a good husband, father, grandfather, an all-around friend to all, and a good patient for all of my doctors.

With the New Year (2015) set to begin in a few short hours, I think it is now time for me to discontinue my writing in this journal. I see no value at this time to put more words on paper just to take up space. If something significant happens to me while I continue on this journey needs to be told, I promise I will let you know.

Epilogue

Although I have halted writing about my day-to-day journey, I will share some of the things I have learned during the past five or six years.

Caregivers

I can't say enough about caregivers, especially **my** caregiver who just happens to be my wife and best friend. I am sure if you would ask her, she would say this just happens to be part of the marriage contract; I guess she is looking at the part that refers to "in sickness and in health." Karen has been by my side at every test and doctor's appointment I have had since my journey with pulmonary fibrosis began. She was with me when I was going through my difficult times during my journey. She was the one sitting in the waiting room as I was going through various procedures during my transplant evaluation. She was the one who took the phone call from Temple on that Sunday morning telling us they had a lung for me and she was the one who waited anxiously for word about how my surgery was progressing. Her smiling face was the first one I saw when I woke up in the ICU. She has been my nurse, my cheerleader, my gopher, my sounding board, my chauffer, my biggest supporter, and as she is fond of saying, she has been my drill sergeant throughout this journey. In my mind, after the role of the transplant surgeon, the caregiver has the most important role in your recovery!

Support Groups

If you are not part of a support group, find one to get involved with. Some hospitals, especially transplant hospitals, have meetings you can attend. Where else can you go and be surrounded by people who are going through the same experiences? There you can talk about how you feel, get answers to questions you have (and God knows you have many questions about this disease) from people who probably have or had some of the same questions you have. The people who attend were once in the same place you are currently in: confused and scared. Most transplant centers, if not all of them, want you as a patient and caregiver to attend these meetings.

Family & Friends

I include family and friends all in the same category. Whether you are part of the immediate family or just friends, you are still considered family in my book. Without all of the offers of help and support that have come our way since this journey began and especially since my transplant, this trip could have been much more difficult for both Karen and me. Just receiving a phone call to say hi or to see if we needed anything has meant so much to both of us.

Family and friends play an important role in this journey, and they will be there for you if and when they are needed.

Humor

I believe if you have read my story, you will note my attempt at humor being infused with seriousness throughout this document. Early on I found out what they have said about humor being a great medicine to be very true. Please don't think I take, or anybody should take, this deadly disease lightly. I chose very early on to not let this disease beat me, and maybe you can say I am laughing in the face of this disease, but it is my way of dealing with pulmonary fibrosis. I have a disease I didn't ask for, and I chose the path I am now following, it is just that I choose not to cry about what happened, but rather smile, laugh and make the best of the situation that has changed my life and changed the lives of those closest to me. Remember the saying that if you laugh, the whole world laughs with you, and if you cry, you cry alone!

It is your choice as to how you proceed on your own journey.

Faith

This is probably the part of my story I shouldn't be talking about, only because of everyone's different take on religion, but for me it was a big part of my journey. I have always believed in God. Have I waivered at times? Absolutely. In my youth, dealing with the death of loved ones, during and after my Vietnam experience, and especially after I was diagnosed with pulmonary fibrosis, my faith probably waivered again. To be honest, each of these experiences, especially the IPF and transplant experience, has probably renewed my faith and made it stronger. I have prayed for guidance as I traveled the road toward transplant; I have prayed for renewed healing strength for myself; I have prayed for the guidance and expertise of the medical staff as they led me down the road toward transplant and for the steady hands of the surgical team who successfully completed my transplant. Does prayer work? I believe absolutely it does! I have said my recovery is in the hands of God and the excellent medical staff looking after my care and recovery.

A word of advice...

No matter where you are on this journey, stay off the Internet, and don't believe everything that is posted is necessarily the truth and applies to your case. You must keep in mind this is where well-meaning people who are on or have been on this journey come together to share their experiences and offer advice as to what may have worked for them; and this is just what it is, their experiences.

This disease affects each of us differently, and as you know there is no cookie cutter cure for IPF. How I am being treated is probably not the same way you are going to be treated. Listen to your doctors, not some well-meaning person who believes his or her treatment is better or worse than what your doctor is prescribing.

Listen to what your doctor is telling you. He or she is the expert. After all that is why he or she is being paid the big bucks. If there is something wrong with you, please don't call me or any other patient for advice. Call your doctor. He or she is the one that is going to be able to help you. All I am going to do is tell you to call your doctor.

Each time I talk to a group or an individual about pulmonary fibrosis, I qualify what I am about to tell them is how this journey or this disease has affected me and not necessarily how it is going to affect them or anybody else.

A final word...

If you have read this entire journal, you have been on my journey with pulmonary fibrosis for almost five years. At this time I continue to recover extremely well from my transplant, and I see no reason why that should not continue. With my continued good health, and if I follow my doctors' orders, I see no reason why I will not be around for many years to come.

I leave you with the following two sayings to think about. I found the following in a magazine, and it sort of sums up this part of my life: Although I still have pulmonary fibrosis, I have a scar you can say is proof of my victory in at least this battle. I haven't won the war, but I will continue to fight until I do.

Never be ashamed of a scar.

Scars are proof of victory.

They simply mean that you were stronger than whatever tried to hurt you.

and

Your life is made of two dates and a dash.

Make the most of that dash.

Peace to all....

Jim

The interpretation of the logo was used with permission of Gift of Life Donor Program. The statements and views expressed in the journal are mine.

Made in the USA
San Bernardino, CA
23 July 2016